Hajrullah Fejza

Virginity, features and concepts in Kosovo Society

AF154896

Hajrullah Fejza

Virginity, features and concepts in Kosovo Society

LAP LAMBERT Academic Publishing

Impressum / Imprint

Bibliografische Information der Deutschen Nationalbibliothek: Die Deutsche Nationalbibliothek verzeichnet diese Publikation in der Deutschen Nationalbibliografie; detaillierte bibliografische Daten sind im Internet über http://dnb.d-nb.de abrufbar.
Alle in diesem Buch genannten Marken und Produktnamen unterliegen warenzeichen-, marken- oder patentrechtlichem Schutz bzw. sind Warenzeichen oder eingetragene Warenzeichen der jeweiligen Inhaber. Die Wiedergabe von Marken, Produktnamen, Gebrauchsnamen, Handelsnamen, Warenbezeichnungen u.s.w. in diesem Werk berechtigt auch ohne besondere Kennzeichnung nicht zu der Annahme, dass solche Namen im Sinne der Warenzeichen- und Markenschutzgesetzgebung als frei zu betrachten wären und daher von jedermann benutzt werden dürften.

Bibliographic information published by the Deutsche Nationalbibliothek: The Deutsche Nationalbibliothek lists this publication in the Deutsche Nationalbibliografie; detailed bibliographic data are available in the Internet at http://dnb.d-nb.de.
Any brand names and product names mentioned in this book are subject to trademark, brand or patent protection and are trademarks or registered trademarks of their respective holders. The use of brand names, product names, common names, trade names, product descriptions etc. even without a particular marking in this works is in no way to be construed to mean that such names may be regarded as unrestricted in respect of trademark and brand protection legislation and could thus be used by anyone.

Coverbild / Cover image: www.ingimage.com

Verlag / Publisher:
LAP LAMBERT Academic Publishing
ist ein Imprint der / is a trademark of
OmniScriptum GmbH & Co. KG
Heinrich-Böcking-Str. 6-8, 66121 Saarbrücken, Deutschland / Germany
Email: info@lap-publishing.com

Herstellung: siehe letzte Seite /
Printed at: see last page
ISBN: 978-3-659-51540-8

Zugl. / Approved by: Orlando, American Academy of Clinical Sexologist, 2013

CONTENT

I. Introduction   2

I.1 Hymen   4

I.2 Literature review   5

I.3 Virginity testing   14

I.4 Statement of the problem   23

II. Aims and objectives of the study   26

III. Research methodology   28

III.2 Study settings   28

III.3 Study methodology   30

III.4 Data collection   30

III.5 Data analysis   31

IV. Hypothesis   32

V. Results   33

V.1 Virginity testing results   33

V.2 Questionnaire results   44

VI. Discussion   52

VII. Conclusions   68

VIII. References   69

I. INTRODUCTION

The word "virginity" first appeared in the 13th century, most frequently in reference to a young woman who has never had sexual intercourse. This does not mean that only heterosexual young women are virgins. Anyone who has never had sex, male or female, can be considered a virgin. Virginity is associated mostly with girls for two reasons. First, virginity traditionally has been, and still is, viewed form society's dominant male and heterosexual perspective. A girl is considered to have lost her virginity only when a male penis has penetrated her. The second reason is because a girl's hymen is ruptured associated with bleeding, which has long been considered proof of intercourse, (*Annie Leah& Michael A. Sommers, 2000*).

Physical health and emotional well-being represent central components of sexual health, according to the World Health Organization (WHO). As defined by the WHO in 2002: Sexual health is a state of physical, emotional, mental and social well-being related to sexuality; it is not merely the absence of disease, dysfunction or infirmity. Sexual health requires a positive and respectful approach to sexuality and sexual relationship, as well as the possibility of having pleasurable and safe sexual experiences, free of coercion, discrimination and violence.

In Kosovo society even today we speak only on female virginity and the requirement to remain virgin until the wedding day.

Throughout human history a women's life was depending on her virginity. A woman who lost virginity before getting married was punished: not honored, her family lost honor, nobody wanted to marry her and in severe cases she was even executed. It did not matter if she lost virginity voluntarily, or if she was raped. Women losing virginity when they were not yet married were denied the right of property. This made their life extremely difficult and as a result many of these women ended up in prostitution.

In some parts of the world, even today there are "honor crimes." Women who lose their virginity before marriage can be beaten or killed by the family. Justification for this is that father, brother or another male relative thinks she has done something "not fair".

According to the "Kanun of Lekë Dukagjini" (a 15th century Law instituted in Northern Albania), which was used by Albanians until the beginning of the 20th century because of lack of state laws," if a girl rejects candidates that have been proposed and there are no mitigating circumstances she must remain a virgin forever".

This Code includes a complex framework of rules, starting from the issues of common concern to the penalties for crimes-some of which this code of law requires the death penalty. Referring to the request for the death penalty for violation of the sexual code, such severe penalties were mostly used in case of sexual relations between blood relatives (incest).

The death penalty does not necessarily apply in cases of loss of virginity. "If it was discovered in the first night of marriage that the woman is not a virgin, she would have been sent back to her family and there" imprisoned "for life, or was forced marry a man from a lower rank of society.

During the past few decades a special attention was paid to female emancipation and the myth about virginity has been changed a lot but the "Kanun of Lekë Dukagjini" and religious norms have prevailed and are still applied in some areas.

I.1 HYMEN

There is a membrane at the vaginal entrance called the hymen. Although people hesitate initially when asked how one can tell whether a woman is a virgin or not, they usually end up remembering the hymen with a relieved smile, (*Anke Bernau, 2007*). During certain periods, gynecological reports declared an unbroken hymen to be a sign of virginity. The hymen is the thin piece of tissue that partly blocks the entrance to the vagina. In many cultures it is serious crime for an unmarried woman to be found with a ruptured hymen, (*Annie Leah& Michael A. Sommers, 2000*).

However, once we accept the definition that virginity could be defined as the absence of any prior sexual intercourse with penetration of the vagina that caused an identifiable lesion of the hymen; we are immediately confronted with a major problem, namely that the integrity of the hymen is not easily assessed! One reason for this is that intact hymens may assume a wide variety of appearances. Depending on the shape and number of its ostia, the hymen is said to be annular (completely encircling the vaginal opening), crescentic (present laterally and posteriorly in the vaginal opening, but deficient in the sub urethral area), septate or cribriform (sieve-like). In rare cases, the hymen may be imperforate; where the complete occlusion of the vaginal orifice leads to retention of the menstrual flow. Congenital absence of the hymen has never been reported. As Rogers3 has stated, the term healed tear (or healed laceration) should only be used when a fresh tear (or laceration) was found in that same area during a previous examination. Superficial notches (less than 50% of the width of the hymeneal rim) are normal findings in non-abused prepubertal girls; notches may likewise have no significance in older females, (*Jean-Jacques Amy, 2007*).

I.2 LITERATURE REVIEW

The term "virgin" was first used in ancient Greece and Rome in reference to a woman who was independent, in the sense that she wasn't the property of any man. It was only later that virginity meant sexual virginity. The most famous virgin is the Virgin Mary, mother of Jesus Christ. She is a central figure in Christianity, and her virginity is of key importance. The impact of 2,000 years of Christianity has left its mark on contemporary Western culture, (*Annie Leah& Michael A. Sommers, 2000*).

If we may judge by appearances, the virginity of the bride played no role in ancient Hellas. This is to explain by the circumstances that in Greece as throughout the east- women and girls were confined to the women's apartment within the house, (*Ottokar Nemecek, 1962*).

During the Middle Ages, there were many ways to test virginity. It was believed that you could detect a virgin by the color of her urine (a virgin's was clear and sparkling) or by the direction in which her breast pointed (a virgin's breast pointed up, toward Heaven), (*Annie Leah& Michael A. Sommers, 2000*).

Saint Augustine in his book "Marriage and Virginity", composed holy virginity as a gift of god, explained how great a gift it is and with what great humility it is to be guarded. Despite his enthusiasm for virginity, however, Augustine spends nearly half of the treatise Holy Virginity in admonitions to the celibate Christian to cultivate the virtue of humility.

The most popular advocate of virginity is the Catholic Church. Its most obvious validation for this stand is the teaching that all young girls are the Virgin Mary's daughters. As such, and having presented Mary as the most pristine and chaste of all women, young Catholic girls are therefore forced to follow her lead throughout their lives. Of course, sex is not prohibited once the woman has entered into the sacrament of marriage. However, while married women are viewed with respect and approval, women who remain virgins all their lives are considered as consecrated. Thus, the latter still achieves a higher status in the Catholic community. Aside from using the Virgin Mary, the Catholic Church has also employed countless symbolisms in order to justify the importance of virginity. Canonizing St. Maria Goretti, who died while trying to fight off a rapist, presents such a symbolism, (*Celeste Ashley, 2005*).

In Both Jewish and Greco-Roman discourse, the virgin is often viewed as a female awaiting marriage. The virgin, nubile and ripe, stands in luminal state. It is in Judaism, especially, that we find such a favorable estimation of marriage that virginity as a prolonged bodily state receives little notice. This was not to suggest that virginity itself was devalued, but rather that virginity was most often viewed as a temporary state in preparation for marriage, an even greater good. One of the tragic consequences of Jepthah's vow is that his daughter dies as a virgin, one who will never wed nor realize her reproductive potential. Virginity was considered in this time as an honor. Virginity yielding only to marriage, the dominant ideal for females in antiquity, presumed a virgin's honor. For the virgin whose social status was inextricably tied to male kin, her sexual status afforded both her and her family honor. The higher bride-price commanded by the Jewish betulah was a monetary expression of honor, *(Mary F. Foskett, 2002).*

The Islamic laws regarding sex are fixed and do not change with peer or siblings pressure or changing the values of the society. Virginity at the time of marriage is considered a virtue in Islamic morality.

In the holy Quran in Appendix 34 is written: "Sons and daughters of the true believers must be taught that their happiness throughout their lives depends on following God's law and preserving their chastity. This means that they must keep themselves for their spouses only, and never allow anyone else to touch them in a sexual manner", (*Quran the Final Testament, by Rashad Khalifa, PhD*). Muslim brides must remain chaste until the night of their wedding. According to Islamic teachings, Allah created the hymen because it serves the function of determining the validity of intercourse, in which women may engage after marriage. The hymen is present in order to make it clear to women that sexual relations outside the marriage bond are perversions of a holy act and are considered unclean. Islam prizes the body's cleanliness above most things, and should, thus, be protected and upheld.

Premarital chastity is still a highly treasured virtue in Hinduism today.

Unlike the modern Western culture, those discussed above maintain the importance of virginity before marriage. However, the decision of whether or not virginity is important depends essentially on personal choice. After all, a woman must be free to choose, without fear or coercion, what she can or cannot do to her own body, *(Celeste Ashley, 2005)*.

Joanne Stroud and Gail Thomas in their book *Images of the Untouched,* published in 1982, described that: "To speak on the part of virginity is to accuse your mothers, which is most infallible disobedience. He that hangs himself is a virgin: virginity murders itself, and should be buried in high-ways, out of all sanctified limit, as a desperate offenders against nature. Virginity breeds mites, much like a cheese, consumes itself to the very paring, and so dies with feeding his own stomach. Besides, virginity is peevish, proud, idle, made of self-love, which is the most inhibited sin in the canon".

John Layard has written the seminal essay sensitizing us to the archetypal psychology of virginity. Virginity, Layard convincingly shows, is a necessity of the soul. It refers neither to absence of nor abstinence form intercourse but rather to the transformation of a basic instinct for union with the mother into a desire for spiritual union with the soul; virginity is a primary telos of the individual soul.

Exploring the problem with an essay entitled" *The taboo of Virginity*"; Freud associated the taboo with the traditional fear of blood, and, by inference, with the more general taboo against murder. Elaborating on the Freud, we can reflect on the potential violence and destructiveness inherent in a virginal mentality, which by definition is untutored in the mores and moral of the civilized life. The reason the husband might fear his virgin wife, says Freud, is first, that she suffers a narcissistic wound with the loss of her physical virginity- she has given up once and for all something valuable and protected; therefore, although she may love her husband, she will also recent his deed. The second, since she has long been deeply attached to her father, or perhaps to a brother, she will be disappointed with her first sexual experience, since her husband can never match her fantasies of love for her father, (*Joanne Stroud and Gail Thomas, 1972*).

Kinsey held that all sex was natural; he argued that the narrow limits prescribed by society were unnatural. Virginity before marriage and sex exclusively within marriage were limited and therefore unnatural-thus, in a sense, immoral, (*Judith A. Reisman & Edward W. Eichel, 1990*).

Carla Stephens, 2003, on her book "*A passion for purity*" wrote: the tokens of virginity are purity, innocence and blood. These tokens act as barriers to negative outside influences that try to inhibit God's plan for your life- for prosperity, hope and a bright future. These three tokens defend you from the enemy's attempts to steal the precious treasure of your virginity. This treasure is often misunderstood or overloaded.

In the same book we can find also that virginity is, indeed, an old concept. In fact, it dates back to biblical times. God, who knows what is best for his creation, presented the concept of virginity to us. We didn't come up with the idea of abstaining from sex before marriage. God did it for our protection and to keep us in union with Him.

The presence or absence of virginity is not measured by how you feel, but it is determined by how you think and what you do with those thoughts.

The headlines as: "A is for Abstinence" (2001), "Choosing Virginity" (2002), "Like a Virgin" (2002), "More in High Schools Are Virgins" (2002), "1 in 5 Teenagers Has sex Before 15' (2003), and " Young Teens and Sex" (2005), are very often in USA. News stories about adolescent sexuality appear in the popular press like clockwork. Almost all of them focus on virginity and virginity loss, the touchstones of American conversations about young people and sex. In some stories, what is news is that teens are losing their virginity; in others, the point is precisely that they're not. More than a few accounts pause to ponder the conflicting ideas those characterize American sexual culture. Nina Bernstein noted in a 2004 New York Times that today's adolescents cannot escape mixed about sex, or the complication of deciding if, when and how to sample it. They are picking form a new multiple-choice menu, where virginity and oral sex can coexist, and erotic rap makes the case for condoms. A lot of interviewed people agreed that a woman or man would lose their virginity the first time they engaged in vaginal sex, provided that they had not previously engaged in another type of genital sex. They also agreed that virginity loss had to involve at least some sort of genital contact between two people. Virginity loss accordingly came to be understood as a rite of passage through which boys were transformed into men and girls into women, *(Laura M. Carpenter, 2005)*.

Making a virginity pledge appears to be an effective means of delaying sexual intercourse initiation among those inclined to pledge without influencing other sexual behavior; pledging does not appear to affect sexual safety among pledges who fail to remain abstinent, *(Martino SC et al. 2008)*

The sexual behavior of virginity pledges does not differ from that of closely matched non-pledges, and pledges are less likely to protect themselves from pregnancy and disease before marriage. Virginity pledges may not affect sexual behavior but may decrease the likelihood of taking precautions during sex, *(Rosenbaum JE, 2009)*

Experiencing less guilt at first sexual intercourse was also strongly associated with psychological satisfaction for women. Developing sexual relationships with partners they care for and trust will foster satisfaction among young people at first vaginal intercourse, *(Higgins JA et al. 2010)*. Significant differences exist in youths' definitions of abstinence and virginity. This suggests that additional attention is needed to ensure a common understanding of these terms to achieve successful sexual education and prevention programs, *(Bersamin MM et al, 2007)*.

Although previous research has found that sexually active teens are more likely to suffer from depression, it is not clear whether this association is causal or spurious in nature. The data from the National Longitudinal Study of Adolescent Health where examined whether virginity status affects self-esteem and depression. For males, fixed effects and instrumental variables (IV) estimates provide little evidence that sex is causally related to psychological well-being. In contrast, IV estimates indicate that sexually active female adolescents are at increased risk of exhibiting the symptoms of depression relative to their counterparts who are not sexually active, (*Sabia JJ, Rees DI, 2008*).

In a study conducted with young women of Maghrebine origin in France show that norms of virginity represent a central means by which women negotiate Maghrebine-French identity and handle intergenerational relations. From the legacy of the colonial era to the current interethnic context, notions of virginity have played a significant role, in both official French discourse, and in the parental transmission of social values across generations. Standards of virginity stand as symbolic markers of women's identity positioning. Yet, women also reinterpret, transform and appropriate codes of virginity according to life experience and situational context, (*Skandrani S et al, 2010*).

The Jewish, Christian and Muslim faiths all attach considerable importance to premarital virginity, particularly that of women. Yet, the social valorization of virginity dates back to a much earlier time than the imposition of chastity upon unmarried women in Muslim communities. Neither the Koran nor Hadiths state that virginity is a precondition to marriage.

Patriarchal societies aim to control the sexuality of women in order to regulate lines of descent and transfer. Islam has only translated a social into a religious norm. It is worth remembering that until the 1960s, moral and behavioral norms kept even European atheists from engaging in premarital sex.

These constraints have only been gradually lifted in the last 50 years as a result of the liberalization of sexuality and the improved social status of women, (*Jean-Jacques Amy, 2008*).

Katha Pollit in her book "Virginity or Death", wrote that there are circulating some ideas to vaccinate women's with a vaccine which can protect from a serious gynecological cancer. Wouldn't that be great? This is refused by Bridget Maher with statement that giving the HPV vaccine to young women could be potentially harmful because they may see it as a license to engage in premarital sex. What is keeping girls virgin now is the threat of getting cervical cancer in midlife from a disease they've probably never heard of, (*Katha Pollit, 2006*)

In his article on "The Taboo of Virginity" (1918), Sigmund Freud describes virginity as a stat notable not primarily for its physical characteristics, but for the psychological turmoil that ensues when a woman 'loses' it. He argues that at the point of first penetrative intercourse the woman experience hostile bitterness against the man, due to her penis envy, which never disappears in the relations between the sexes. Virginity for religious writers in the twentieth and twenty-first centuries, as for their predecessors, is both a physical and a spiritual state. An alternative to this view of virginity- men is founded in some writings on virginity, "mainly by women", in which virginity allows them to escape the demands imposed by a male-dominated society. Frequently, this is also linked to the idea that virginity becomes the primary and positive precondition for women's writing. A virgin daughter did not only act as a mirror of her father's ability to control his family affairs; she could be a valuable asset in his economic and political dealings. As we can see, the value of virginity was viewed very differently within the religious and the secula spheres, (*Anke Bernau, 2007*)

I.3 VIRGINITY TESTING

In Kosovo, although prohibited by law in 2002, virginity testing is still performed at the Institute of Forensic Medicine in Prishtina. This testing is carried by the commission, which includes gynecologist and medical forensic specialist. The prohibition of this testing for many years led to great pressure from stakeholders to determine virginity in order to resolve problems dealing with marriage, with violations, rape and for testimony before marriage. As a result of this, the Institute performs this test on request by interested people and issues a certificate which parties can use for their own purposes. This testing in any case is not bound by anyone including the Court and the prosecution which until 2002 had been actors in this kind of testing. The circumstances under which the virginity test is requested are different and range from women who insist on doing this test on a voluntary basis, partner's request, sometimes done with the insistence of parents and in some cases after rape or attempted rape. Given the historical, cultural and religious circumstances, Kosovo society has advanced significantly in this regard and cases that seek to solve problems through virginity test are very low.

Kosovo has been occupied by Ottoman Empire for many centuries and these left visible traces in the religious aspect which has greatly impacted the perception of sex and virginity among people in this area.

At the same time the "Kanun of Lekë Dukagjini" has also been very strict in relation to sex and virginity, making it even harder for non-virgin girls to live a normal life.

After the Kosovo war of 1999, with the arrival of many foreigners and soldiers in our country starts an overall revolution and a great opening to the European civilization, including sexual freedom which until this time was very unfavorable for Kosovo women. Now, more and more electronic media and magazines talk about sex and the inevitable theme is virginity as a problem which for centuries has affected the female population. Now there is increasing number of young people to whom the virginity of their female partner is not of prime interest which in its way represents a kind of sexual revolution.

Virginity testing - Literature review

A virginity test is the practice and process of inspecting the genitalia of girls and women to determine if they are sexually chaste. It is based on the false assumption that a woman's hymen can only be torn as a result of sexual intercourse.

The world is characterized by the conflict existing between human rights and customary practices. Customary laws and practices appear to be in major and difficult conflict to harmonize. It differs from country to country as to one must be applied when the two are in conflict or contrary to each other. Virginity testing is one of the practices which grab a lot of attention in conflicting with human rights from country to country. The harmonization of customary laws and human rights is not given the attention it seeks by authors around the world, *(T.G. Ramatsekisa, 2010)*

Yet the hymen is a more elusive membrane than is commonly assumed, and its status as sure sign of virginity is in fact doubtful. An article in Lancet in 1978 stated that: "Contrary to popular belief no definite criteria have ever been established for deciding whether a woman is a virgin or not", and that therefore "it is extremely difficult for the medical examiner to state with certainty whether the woman is, or not, a virgin'. The authoritative tone of this statement demonstrates the persistence of the idea that female virginity is indeed physically verifiable, even visible and concrete. Female virginity becomes a universally accepted condition, one that needs not to be thought about further. This assumption is usually based on the hymen, whose presence or absence becomes central to a woman's sexual and social identity, as well as her self-understanding, *(Anke Bernau, 2007)*

Virginity testing is done in different ways, depending upon the country. Primarily, the vagina is examined to see whether or not the girl's hymen is intact. The hymen is defined as "the thin membrane of skin that may stretch across part of the vaginal opening". The opening of the hymen allows the menstruation to flow out of the body.

Most girls are born with a hymen, although some are born without it. Many doctors say that the hymen is not a good indicator of sexual virginity for several reasons:

(1) A girl may have been born without a hymen;

(2) The hymen can easily be ruptured during normal physical activities and sports;

(3) The hymen can be stretched open by the use of tampons.

Often the bed sheet from a couple's wedding night is examined to see if any blood is present on it because a virgin is supposed to bleed during her first sexual encounter. However, a woman may be a virgin and still not bleed during her first intercourse, (*T.G. Ramatsekisa, 2010*).

Virginity testing has become a relatively new trend in many countries; especially those are highly concerned with women's honor and infectious diseases such as HIV/AIDS. Females of all ages (ranging from as young as 4 months to 50 years) essentially queue up and have their vaginas inspected to see if their hymens are intact. If they are, the women are found to be virgins. In South Africa, the practice has become more common in recent years. The motivation behind the revival of this testing comes from concern amongst traditional leaders about the increasing prevalence of HIV/AIDS. It is believed that this testing promotes abstinence and curtails the spread of HIV/AIDS among the youth.

Virginity testing is also seen as a way of curbing women sexual activity before marriage and keeping them "pure" until then. There are many controversies and debates as to whether or not this infringes upon women's human rights, even if they participate willingly, (*T.G. Ramatsekisa, 2010*).

In most African countries the virginity testing is initiated for HIV and other Sexually transmitted diseases. In the absence of effective measures against AIDS, inhabitants try to find alternative ways to protect young people. An older tradition that emphasizes the status of virgin girls and the significance of the collective is used in a strategy that incorporates HIV blood tests. Virginity testing is a 'preventive ritual' more than a 'diagnostic measure', while emphasizing how both South African and Western projects aimed at improving the situation are grounded in perspectives that sometimes collide with how local people conceive of both relationships and sexuality,(*Wickström, A,2010*).

About 120,000 South Africans in 2005 were estimated to have died of HIV/AIDS-related illnesses and more than 100,000 HIV/AIDS orphans have been created. This has made community leaders extremely interested in reviving the old cultural tradition of virginity testing as a way to safeguard against HIV/AIDS. They believe that by testing for virginity, they are protecting themselves by telling people to abstain from sex. These examinations have become extremely popular and hundreds of girls wait in line for up to three hours to be tested, (*T.G. Ramatsekisa, 2010*)

Umhlanga is a ceremony celebrating virginity. In South Africa, it is practiced, among others, by the Zulu ethnic group who live mainly in the province of

KwaZulu Natal. After falling into relative disuse in the Zulu community, the practice of virginity testing made a comeback some 10 years ago at around the time of the country's first democratic election and coinciding with the period when the HIV pandemic began to take hold. In July 2005 the South African Parliament passed a new Children's Bill which will prohibit virginity testing of children, (*Vincent L, 2006*).

In India there is a centuries-old custom of Kukariki Rasam (thread ritual), where a skein of thread is used to detect the presence of an intact hymen. It isn't just used to torture women, but is often used so that the bride's family can make money. "Impure" brides are beaten to reveal the names of their "lovers" and then these lovers are forced to pay large amounts of money to the bride's family. Under the pain of torture, Sansi women suspected of fornication often name any man that they know just to stop the torture that they are undergoing. Virginity tests are not covered in the Indian Criminal Code and therefore cannot be considered a crime, so procedure cannot be filed against these practices. Women's organizations in India are active, but the movement to end virginity testing is not strong as of yet. Other tests used in India are the Paaniki Dheej (purity by water) or Agnipariksha (trial by fire), (*T.G. Ramatsekisa, 2010*).

Solomon Rothman, in 2005 wrote an article about virginity testing in Turkey and there is shown as follows: In the mostly Muslim culture of Turkey, it's a social norm for females to remain virgins until marriage. Female virginity is not only highly valued, it's expected. Virginity is celebrated and is symbolic of the woman's importance as mother of the home and of how her body belongs only to her husband. This belief is so emphasized in the Turkish culture, that it's a normal cultural practice to test a female's virginity, even against her will. This is done for many reasons including, verifying the virginity of a potential bride, certifying that sexual relations did not occur prior to marriage, suspicion of consensual sexual intercourse, and lack of vaginal bleeding after first marital intercourse. Unmarried females found not to be virgins experience great shame and legal discrimination. Proof of un-chastity is a valid reason for the permanent expulsion of females from the formal educational system. A female that is found to not be a virgin is labeled unfit to marry by most of the society. The shame is so great that there have been many reports of girls committing suicide before such a test.

On 19 July 2001, the Minister of Health of Turkey initiated proceedings to bypass the ban on virginity examinations (Ministry of Justice, decree no: 27/123) brought into action two years ago after many years of protest by women and women's groups in Turkey. Turkey's health minister says high school girls training to be nurses must be virgins and the virginity tests he is authorizing will protect the nation's youth from prostitution and underage sex. Outraged women's groups and nurses are vowing to fight, and a teachers' union is asking the government to fire the minister. In Turkey, girls who attend nursing high schools are generally from poor, traditional backgrounds. The conservative countryside is a traditional power base for Durmus' far-right Nationalist Action Party. The 1999 ban on virginity tests allows them only for gathering evidence for court cases, such as rape trials. It requires a court order before women can be forced to take the test, (*Women for Women's Human Rights/ Kadinin Insan Halklari Projesi, 2001*).

Hamila Nisgeleli, in Rozahen Magazine said that in the Islamic Republic of Iran according to custom women must go a virgin on her marriage bed. This expectation is so "obvious" and "natural" that it does not appear anywhere in print. Neither in the *sharia'* nor the Civil Code will you find virginity as a pre-condition for marriage or for its dissolution. It does not appear in any legal document. But this "law" runs deep in social psychology and has imposed endless tragedies. Yet the man is not expected to be a virgin. Indeed sexual experience before marriage is considered in some ways necessary.

Girls are forced to experience their first sexual encounter on the marriage bed. That first night is turned into a night of fear and dread, an examination on which her future depends. Not only she is denied the chance of enjoying her first encounter with this form of human relation, but in practice it overshadows in her mind everything else in her new shared life. From childhood girls are forbidden many sports and games. Yet the fear that she may have jumped too high here, or ran too fast there, haunts her on the wedding night. During the ceremony she had to bear the anxious and questioning looks of her immediate relatives.

The custom of obtaining a medical certificate to prove the virginity of the woman and handing it to the family of the groom, which prevailed earlier among certain urban layers in Iran, was fast becoming isolated and unacceptable. With the Islamic Republic it has not only spread among urban society but even penetrated educated and "modern" layers.

Progressive and revolutionary forces, with claims to change or overturn society, not only failed to question this custom, but were themselves firm adherents. This shows the true extent of the catastrophe and signifies the depth of misogyny in society. The "law" of virginity is so deep, and so unquestionable that an overwhelming majority fail to notice it, let alone question it. The frightening dimension of the violence and debasement of women concealed in it is thus ignored.

More than 150 women have been examined at the forensic medical institutions in the capital Amman, and in the North and South of the country of Jordan during the last year, according to official records. The unofficial figures might be higher due to the fact that some newly-wed brides are taken straight to private gynecology clinics, or to midwives. Private records of midwife Huda Al Zagha, who worked from 1941 to 2000, have shown that she examined 30 women throughout her work experience. All exams took place with the women's consent, based on the request of the husband, the parent, judicial authorities or clan elders, (*Arab reporters for Investigative Journalism*).

Win (2004) argues that in Kenya virginity testing helps to delay the age at first sex among rural Kenyan youth and it reduces vulnerability to sexually transmitted infections and HIV infections. Hunter (1936) argues that virginity testing is done in order to ensure that girls who are virgins have much broader significance. Virgins are seen as morally pure and more important because they are able to maintain their virginity up until marriage. Engaging in sexual intercourse before marriage is not acceptable, (*Sithembile Promise Mhlongo*).

According to the media, doctors in several European countries are increasingly asked by young women, mostly but not exclusively of Muslim faith, to deliver certificates of virginity to them and to reconstruct their hymens. It is estimated that a few hundreds of these certificates are now delivered annually in Belgium.

The inspection of the hymen is thus frequently unrevealing with regard to the sexual history of the woman concerned. Submitting her for the benefit of others to the examination of her genitals for the purpose of ascertaining her chastity is a transgression of her intimacy and an insult to her dignity. The examination is so unreliable, that the certificate of 'virginity' – supposedly written after completion of the said examination – should be considered devoid of any objective value, (*Jean-Jacques Amy, 2008*)

I.4 STATEMENT OF THE PROBLEM

Virginity as a concept in most countries of Western Europe and the U.S. remains as "old fashion", but in some countries of Africa, Asia, South America and South-Eastern Europe continues to be taboo and bring numerous problems for women who lose it before marriage.

Kosovo, as the region became part of the countries of South-East Europe, populated by the majority Muslim Albanians and therefore the impact of culture, tradition and religion in terms of sex and virginity still continues to be great.

The fact that in Kosovo society publicly is very little spoken about sex, pleasures and consequences of its absence prompted us to believe that any study which is aimed at researching the facts and opinions about sexual life in this sense also for virginity will have great benefit to society, especially for women who in large part continue to suffer the consequences of patriarchal society, local behavior and habits.

The combination of culture, tradition and religion in this region is very influential in the sexual life of the population. In some rural areas population lives and acts according to the "Kanun of Lekë Dukagjini" which is rigorous in tackling problems that arise from extramarital sexual activities. The influence of religion and religious clerics who through daily discourses significantly affect the deeper concepts and differences between those who believe blindly towards the part of the population which tends to emancipate and exceeds the old beliefs and attitudes.

Faced with this reality, many young people find themselves at a crossroad of whether to respect tradition and religion in their lives or to make selection according to his will and mind as do their peers around the world. Not a small number of young people who select the mode of living differently from parents and family are forced to leave their family. But there are those who due to the influence of family and circumstances give up from their love just because of the virginity.

The concept of virginity in Kosovo deals on female virginity only. A non- virgin woman on the first night of marriage if not accepted normal from her husband shall be sent back to the family and cannot ever marry a bachelor. In most cases she is forced to marry someone much older or a widowed man.

Kosovo schools still do not teach anything about sex education and in most family's sex and virginity are a taboo. Young people in our society entering puberty and experiencing their sexual fantasies are unprepared and everything they learn is on the hand of fate and what they can get from their peers, magazines or other media.

This concept and these contradictions in the Kosovo society make this problem very serious. The findings of this study will show us whether we are still as a society with an old-fashioned mentality or there are signs that a change has begun which will give hope that the determinant of the fate for women life's in Kosovo will not be virginity but the character and her commitment to love and being loved.

During the presentation and explanation of this topic to the professors and colleagues of the American Academy for Clinical Sexologist there were different objections and reactions from them because they couldn't believe that in this society virginity still has an important role in the lives of young people, especially for the women. Wishing to tackle this taboo theme it was decided to do an analysis and research among different levels of young kosovars.

II. AIMS AND OBJECTIVES OF THE STUDY

The overall objective of the study was to explore perceptions of virginity and virginity testing in Kosovo society in total and among young people in particular. The study will be significant in the following ways. Firstly, the study will provide a deeper understanding of virginity from the perspective of young adolescents and draw on different arguments put forward by the people who think that virginity is still very important and virginity testing should continue and people who feel that it should be banned. Secondly, the study will expand the literature on virginity and virginity testing. The study looks at both the importance and implications of this practice.

There is a belief that in Kosovo there are major contradictions and differences about virginity which are dealing with the question of whether there is still value being a virgin.

In this study it was attempted to find answers to some questions, like:

• Is female virginity pre-condition to enter into marriage?

• What are the consequences of losing virginity before marriage?

• Is virginity test still tool to determine the fate of marriages?

• Are young people willing to marry a non-virgin partner?

The study was focused on the analysis of virginity tests which are still used as a tool to solve problems relating to marriage, pre marital agreements and dispute resolution between different pairs, on the one hand, and through an administered questionnaire among students on the other side.

Implications of cultural, religious, living conditions and education would be treated with special care being convinced that there are major differences in this aspect.

All findings from this study will be compared with the relevant literature and will be discussed thoroughly trying to find the place for Kosovo society in this area which is very sensitive and important for young people.

III. RESEARCH METHODOLOGY

III.1. Introduction

The epidemiological descriptive study method with retrospective and prospective analysis would be used in this research using mixed qualitative methods: virginity testing certificate analysis and self-administered questionnaire.

III.2. Study Setting

III.2.1 Kosovo

Kosovo is the youngest country in the world. The independence is declared on 17 February 2008. The state is landlocked and borders Serbia north and eastward, the Republic of Macedonia to the south, Albania to the west and Montenegro to the northwest (the latter three recognize it as independent). The largest city and the capital of Kosovo is Prishtina. Kosovo represents an important link between central and southern Europe and the Adriatic and Black Seas. Kosovo has an area of 10,908 square km. Its climate is continental, with warm summers and cold and snowy winters. According to the Kosovo in Figures 2005 Survey of the Statistical Office of Kosovo the total population is estimated between 1.9 and 2.2 million with the following ethnic composition: Albanians

92%, Serbs 4%, Bosniaks and Gorans 2%, Turks 1%, Roma 1%. The two predominant languages of Kosovo are Albanian and Serbian. The two main religions of Kosovo are Islam and Christianity. Muslims make up 90% of Kosovo's population and followers are mostly Sunni, with a Bektashi Islam minority.

Figure .1 Kosovo in a Balkan map

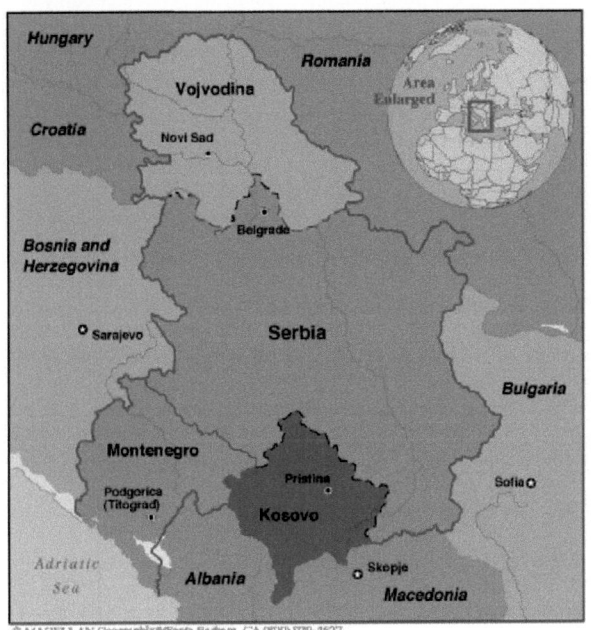

III. 3   STUDY METHODOLOGY

Retrospective study concerns the analysis of virginity tests analyzing different variables dealing with age, occupation, residence, reason for testing and the conclusion of the screening committee. Prospective research consists in developing self-administered questionnaire prepared specially for this research. The quality of collected data will be checked during all stages of research: the stage of collecting data about completing the form, consistency and quality at the point of data entry during the purification and analysis. These security level of data quality, ensure that the results obtained are of acceptable quality.

III.4   DATA COLLECTION

Data for virginity test are collected from the Institute of Forensic Medicine of Kosovo with the prior approval and confidentiality declaration.

The period of analysis covers the years after the Kosovo war between the period times 2000-2010. The data from a cross-sectional survey on concepts about the virginity comes from students of Public University of Prishtina and one from a Private University College in Kosovo carried out in 2011. Data for this study was collected from 296 male students and 232 female students. Due to the sensitive nature of the study, a self-administrated structured questionnaire was used to obtain information from the students. The questionnaires were first developed in English and then translated into Albanian language.

III.5 DATA ANALYSIS

All completed survey questionnaires and reports from virginity testing were entered into a database after manual coding and validation. Data entry and validity checks were performed for all the questionnaires by using computer software dBase IV. The cleaned and validated data was transferred into SPSS (Statistical Package for Social Sciences, Version 13, SPSS Inc., Chicago, IL), for further processing and analysis. Chi-square test was used to test an association between the variables.

Verbal informed consent was obtained from the participants before they were enrolled in the study. Consent form was written in the local language stating the study's objectives, nature of participant's involvement, risk and benefits, and confidentiality of the data. Students were requested to read the consent form carefully. They were given clear options on voluntary participation. It was also made clear that they could refuse to answer any questions and terminate the interview when they desired. None of the approached students refused to participate in the study. Confidentiality of information was provided by removing personal identifiers from the completed questionnaires. The names of sampled colleges were not made public and thus not possible for anyone outside the research team to trace reported incidents of sexual behaviour to respondents. Respondents were protected from any possible adverse repercussions of participating in the study.

IV. HYPOTHESIS

Ho- virginity is still the determining factor for marriage and still virginity test is the tool to determine the fate of marriages in a part of Kosovo society.

H1- virginity is not the determining factor for marriage and virginity test is not the tool to determine the fate of marriages in Kosovo society.

V. RESULTS

In order to fulfill the objectives of the study we included two types of surveys that include different study populations with quite different mentalities and features from each other.

The first part of this chapter describes results of research dealing with the virginity test while the second part presents the results of the survey conducted with students.

V.1 Virginity testing results

Reports from virginity testing (544) collected from Institute of Forensic Medicine in Prishtina were analyzed from which are derived the most important variables that help us to test our hypothesis about the features and concepts of virginity in Kosovo.

General characteristics show that age group with most represent cases was between 25-29 years with a total of 181 cases or 33.3%. It is important to notice that 3 cases were aged less than 10 years which made the test by the family insistence after their suspicion that they could have lost virginity in different situations which are not described in detail in the report.

We have analyzed the occupation of women who underwent the test to determine which category is represented by more cases in this study. However, not all (30%) have declared their occupation while the unemployed women lead with 38.6%.

The civil status of women who underwent virginity testing was: 64.9% unmarried, 18% married while 16% engaged, (Table 1).

Table 1 General characteristics of the study population

Age	Frequency	Percent
Under 10 y.	3	0.6
10-14y	4	0.7
15-19	17	3.1
20-24	151	27.8
25-29	181	33.3
30-34	114	21
35-39	34	6.3
40-44	7	1.3
No data	33	6.1
Total	544	100
Occupation	Frequency	Percent
unemployed	210	38.6
teacher	7	1.3
child	27	5
hairdresser	6	1.1
nurse	1	0.2
jurist	1	0.2
pupils	69	12.7
police	2	0.4
worker	20	3.7
student	38	7
no data	163	30
Total	544	100
Civil status	Frequency	Percent
engaged	87	16
married	98	18
maiden	353	64.9
no data	6	1.1
Total	544	100

Residency of women and their partners has been the object of study because we suspect that our society still has major differences in social concepts between urban and rural areas having in mind patriarchal families and the impact of religion and culture in this issue. Of the total number of women who have done the test, 59.4% are from rural areas and 31.6% of male partners of women who are subjected to the test come from rural areas, (Table 2).

Table 2   The residence of study population

	Female		Mail	
Residence	Frequency	Percent	Frequency	Percent
rural	323	59.4	172	31.6
urban	200	36.8	97	17.8
no data	21	3.9	275	50.6
Total	544	100.0	544.0	100.0

p<o.o5

This suspicion was strengthened further by analyzing the reasons that have driven women to do the virginity test and we found that of 323 rural women, 119 cases have made the test due to suspicion of partner and only 55 from the urban areas, 75 of them did the test to confirm their virginity and 47 underwent virginity test by prosecutor order, (Table 3).

Table 3 Relationship between the female residency and reasons for virginity test

Reason for testing	Female residency			Total
	Rural	urban	no data	
rape	1	1	0	2
partner doubt	119	55	0	174
doubt on hymenoplasty	1	0	0	1
family insistence	20	15	3	38
prosecutor order	52	47	4	103
own insistence	75	46	1	122
confirmation	3	4	0	7
injury	4	4	2	10
police order	47	26	11	84
social worker order	1	2	0	3
Total	323	200	21	544

Even in the case of the male partner residency the same situation is observed. A total of 101 out of 171 male subjects which asked their female partners to perform the test due to their doubt were from rural areas, while 51 of them were from urban areas (Table 4).

Table 4 Relationship between the male residency and reasons for virginity test

Reason for testing	Male residency			Total
	rural	urban	no data	
rape	1	0	2	2
partner doubt	101	51	22	174
doubt on hymenoplasty	0	1	0	1
family insistence	2	2	34	38
prosecutor order	4	0	98	103
own insistence	51	34	37	122
confirmation	0	1	6	7
injury	1	0	9	10
police order	11	8	65	84
social worker order	0	0	3	3
Total	171	97	276	544

One other variable that we analyzed from virginity testing has been the frequency of sexual intercourse of women before they went for testing. We found that 42.6% had only one sexual intercourse, 14.5% more than one sexual intercourse while 3.9% did not have any sexual intercourse, (Table 5).

Table 5   Frequency of sexual intercourses before virginity testing

Nr of sexual intercourses	Frequency	Percent
0	21	3.9
1	232	42.6
1+	79	14.5
no data	212	39.0
Total	544	100.0

Interesting data are extracted from the test reports or medical committee conclusion. From overall number, in 52.2% of cases hymen was intact, 22.8% had a fresh broken hymen and 22.6% had an old broken hymen. In 9 cases it was impossible testing because of lack of cooperation of women, (Table 6).

Table 6 Results (conclusions) after the virginity test

Results	Frequency	Percent
fresh broken hymen	124	22.8
intact	284	52.2
no cooperation	9	1.7
hymenoplasty	1	0.2
old broken hymen	123	22.6
no data	3	0.6
Total	544	100

Interesting results we found after analyzing the relationship between the frequency of sexual relations and test results.

In total of 544 cases analyzed more than half of the results, 284 cases have shown that the hymen has been intact, fresh broken hymen were in 124 cases and in 123 cases were with old broken hymen.

It is interesting that in 31 cases who have had sexual intercourse more than once hymen has been intact. In 4 cases there was a declaration that they have never had sexual intercourse, yet hymen was old broken, (Table 7).

Table 7   Relationship between frequency of coitus and test results

Test result	Frequency of coitus				Total
	0	1	1+	no data	
fresh broken hymen	1	77	25	21	124
intact	16	103	31	134	284
malformation	0	0	1	0	1
no cooperation	0	4	0	5	9
hymenoplasty	0	0	0	1	1
old broken hymen	4	47	22	50	123
no data	0	1	0	1	2
Total	21	232	79	212	544

When analyzed the reasons why women undergo virginity test we found that number of women who undergo testing ordered by the prosecutor is 84 or 15.5% of cases.

After the 2002 virginity testing were done at the insistence of the parties for the purpose of resolving conflicts between the partners and their families. In this period we have 32% of cases when the test is done with the insistence of a doubtful partner.

A phenomenon which has resulted in significant number of cases in this analysis has also been testing with own insistence in order of confirmation of virginity. Of the total number, 22.4% have undergone testing only to confirm whether they are virgins or not and 18.9% with own insistence, without specifying the exact cause of testing. The role of family in all this analysis has not been small because 7% of cases have made test at the behest of family, (Table 8).

Table 8   The reason why the test was done

Reason	Frequency	Percent
rape	2	0.4
partner doubt	174	32
doubt on hymenoplasty	1	0.2
family insistence	38	7
prosecutor order	84	15.5
own insistence	103	18.9
confirmation	122	22.4
injury	7	1.3
police order	10	1.8
social worker order	4	0.6
Total	544	100

Suspicion of the partner as a main reason to force women to perform the test is shown to be non-reasonable by the fact that of 174 cases only 30 of them presented with old broken hymen, hymen had been intact in 76 cases while in 68 cases hymen was fresh broken. Even in the case of testing after family insistence, hymen has been intact in 32 out of 38 cases. Interestingly, the outcome in cases where women underwent testing at their own will for confirmation purpose, out of 122 such cases, 28 had fresh broken hymen, 24 cases had old broken hymen and in 67 cases the hymen was intact, (Table 9).

Table 9 Relationship between the reason of testing and results

| Reason | Result | | | | | | |
	fresh broken hymen	intact	no cooperation	Hymeno plasty	no data	old broken hymen	Total
rape	0	2	0	0	0		2
partner doubt	68	76	0	0	0	30	174
doubt on hymenoplasty	0	1	0	0	0	0	1
family insistence	1	32	0	0	1	4	38
prosecutor order	10	33	6	0	0	35	84
own will	11	66	1	1	0	24	103
confirmation	28	67	2	0	1	24	122
injury	2	3	0	0	0	1	7
police order	4	2	0	0	0	4	10
social worker order	0	2	0	0	1	1	4
Total	124	284	9	1	3	123	544

The relationship between civil status of study population and reason which pushes the parties to undergo virginity testing shows interesting results. All cases ordered for testing by order of the prosecutor belongs to the category of women who were not betrothed or married. From this category which includes the largest number of women tested, 96 out of 353 of them have been tested by own will and 75 for the purpose of confirmation the virginity. Of the 98 married women who underwent testing, 74 of them have done test after suspicions of their partner, mainly after the first night of marriage. About 70 % of betrothed women underwent test due to the suspicion expressed by the partner (Table 10).

Table 10 Relation between civil status and reason for virginity test

Reason	Civil status				Total
	maiden	engaged	married	no data	
Rape	2	0	0	0	2
partner doubt	40	60	74	0	174
doubt on hymenoplasty	1	0	0	0	1
family insistence	36	1	0	1	38
own will	96	2	0	5	103
Confirmation	75	24	23	0	122
Injury	6	0	1	0	7
police order	10	0	0	0	10
prosecutor order	84	0	0	0	84
social worker order	3	0	0	0	3
Total	353	87	98	6	544

A comparison of test results with the occupation of the studied population was also done. Studies show that the category of the unemployed and students lead to greater number of three key findings of the medical committee. Of 210 cases of unemployed, 47 were with old broken hymen, 101 of them had intact hymen while in 60 cases hymen was fresh broken. Students are the second largest category represented in this study. By their total number of 163, the old broken hymen have been found in 39 cases, 84 had intact hymen while in 36 cases there was fresh broken hymen.

Throughout this study there was only one case with hymenoplasty and her occupation was police officer, (Table 11).

Table 11 Relation between occupation and results of virginity test

Occupation	fresh broken hymen	intact	no cooperation	hymeno plasty	no data	old broken hymen	Total
			Result				
unemployed	60	101	0	0	2	47	210
teacher	1	3	0	0	0	3	7
child	2	19	3	0	0	3	27
hairdresser	0	4	0	0	0	2	6
nurse	1	0	0	0	0	0	1
lawyer	1	0	0	0	0	0	1
pupils	11	43	2	0	1	12	69
police	0	0	0	1	0	1	2
worker	5	6	0	0	0	9	20
student	36	84	4	0	0	39	163
no data	7	24	0	0	0	7	38
Total	124	284	9	1	3	123	544

V.2 Questionnaire results

In order to obtain opinions about the attitudes among young people in Kosovo about virginity and with the purpose of verifying presented hypothesis, a survey with students of different levels in Prishtina was performed. The survey was conducted in a Public University of Prishtina and in one private University College.

The study included 530 students, of whom 55.8% were male and 43.8% female. Their residency is analyzed in order to research whether there is a role of the origin in their stance on virginity. There have been 50.9% of them coming from urban areas. The 83.9% of participants were in the age group 18-25 years, (Table 12).

Table 12 General characteristics of participants

Gender	Nr	%
M	296	55.8
F	232	43.8
Not known	2	0.4
Total	530	100
Residence		
Urban	270	50.9
Rural	245	46.2
Not known	15	2.8
Total	530	100
Age		
18-25y	445	83.9
26+	68	12.9
Not known	17	3.2
Total	530	100

On the question of whether virginity is still taboo in Kosovo, from a total of 503 respondents, 340 cases responded with positive answer.

Those results do not differ much in the answers given by both sexes. The difference between the sexes on this issue is very small, 65% women and 63% males, (Table 13).

Table 13   Virginity is still a taboo?

		Taboo			
		Yes	No	Don't know	Total
Gender	M	187	64	45	296
	F	151	45	36	232
	Not known	2	0	0	2
Total		340	109	81	530

For further elaboration on the importance of virginity issue, another question related to whether there is an advantage to being a virgin in Kosovo was also submitted and again there was positive response from both genders. The total number of those who think it is an advantage was 350 out of 530 respondents. No significant difference in response between the sexes was observed, (Table 14).

Table 14 Virginity is an advantage

		Virginity is an advantage			
		Yes	No	Don't know	Total
Gender	M	195	81	20	296
	F	154	57	21	232
	Not known	1	1	0	2
Total		350	139	41	530

P<0.05

When they were asked if it is the same importance between male and female virginity, by the total number of 530 respondents, 371 cases or 70% answered no. The difference between males and females in this question is too small, and there is no statistical significance, (Table 15).

Table 15   Female and male virginity has a same importance

		Same importance			
		Yes	No	Don't know	Total
Gender	M	66	202	28	296
	F	38	168	26	232
	Not known	1	1	0	2
Total		105	371	54	530

The next variable analyzed the responses of students in terms of virginity as a prerequisite for marriage. A total of 334 out of 530 cases responded positively. There is no difference between genders either in this case, (Table 16).

Table 16 Virginity is prerequisite for marriage

		Prerequisite			
		Yes	No	Don't know	Total
Gender	M	179	82	35	296
	F	155	51	26	232
	Not known	1	1	0	2
Total		334	135	61	530

p<0.05

A very interesting phenomenon has emerged by the answers given to the following question: are you virgin? It is interesting that although all questions have been answered earlier that virginity is more important, that it is a prerequisite for marriage, etc., the number of those who stated that they are not virgin is 296 out of 530 or 56%, which is much larger compared with those who declare themselves as virgins. However, there is statistically significant difference between the sexes. Of the total 232 women surveyed 142 or 61.20% of them declare themselves as virgins, compared to men where only 17.9% state that they are virgins. This finding proves once again that there is significant difference between male and female virginity and significantly larger number of women keep their virginity until marriage. This probably speaks best to the concept of Kosovo society on virginity and the role of tradition and family in this issue, (Table 17).

Table 17 Are you virgin?

		Are you virgin			
		Yes	No	No answer	Total
Gender	M	53(17.9%)	214(72.30%)	29(9.8%)	296(100.0%)
	F	142(61.20%)	82(35.30)	8(3.5%)	232(100.0%)
	Not known	1	0	1	2
Total		196(37%)	296(56%)	38(7%)	530(100.0%)

$$p<0.05$$

Another interesting answer that actually isn't in line with those who speak of the great importance of virginity is the finding that 249 cases of total 530 would marry a non - virgin partner. Here, the difference between the sexes is very big. While 63.7% of women said they could marry non-virgin partners, this is accepted by 33% of men. This actually explains the positive answers given by subjects in total when asked about the importance of virginity, and also speaks about the fact stated earlier that male virginity is not as important as virginity of a female, (Table 18).

Table 18   Would you get married with a non virgin partner?

		Get married with not virgin partner			
		Yes	No	Don't know	Total
Gender	M	99	121	76	296
	F	148	52	32	232
	Not known	1	1	0	2
Total		249(63.7%)	173(33.0%)	108(20.3%)	530(100.0%)

p<0.05

The next two questions were only for men and had to do with virginity test made at the request of interested parties. When asked if after suspicion on virginity they would ask the partner to undergo the test, 170 or 48% of men participating in the study answered yes, while 126 or 42% said no, (Table 19).

Table 19   Is a doubt about virginity reason to ask for test?

Ask for test	Frequency	Percent
Yes	126	42.0
No	170	48.0
Total male	296	100.0

While on the question of whether virginity test showing that the partner is not a virgin will result in divorce, 124 or 42% of cases answered with YES, 122 or 41% gave negative answer, while 50 cases or 17% have stated that they wouldn't know how to act, (Table 20).

Table 20   If the test shows a female is not virgin would you ask for divorce?

Divorce	Frequency	Percent
Yes	124	42.0
No	122	41.0
Don't know	50	17.0
Total male	296	100.0

In the last question dealing with a relatively widespread phenomenon in Kosovo which has to do with hymen repair or hymenoplasty both sexes stated that they are against this action as a measure to present a false virginity. Of the total number of 530 cases, 356 declared that it is not the right action while only 65 or 12.5% of cases declared hymenoplasty as a right action, (Table 21).

Table 21   Hymenoplasty is right action

		Hymenoplasty right action?			
		Yes	No	Don't know	Total
Gender	M	31	230	62	296
	F	34	152	46	232
	Not known	0	1	1	2
Total		65	356	109	530

In none of our questions in survey there were differences in response between the cases that came from the urban and rural area.

VI. DISCUSSION

Although in most Western countries the issue of virginity is irrelevant and has no role in society or among young people who are entering in relationship or prior to marriage, in Kosovo, having in mind the circumstances and concepts of society, the influence of family, culture and religion the topic of female virginity has been barely discussed, while in most cases it is a prerequisite for durable and successful marriage.

Virginity has become an obsolete concept in modern Western society, allowing young women to experiment with their sexuality while their male counterparts are doing the same. This actually results in a healthier more well-adjusted sexual identity later in life. However, virginity has not totally left the modern scene. Many cultures are still upholding the value of virginity or pre-marital chastity, mainly on the basis of predominant religious concepts. The most popular advocate of virginity is the Catholic Church. Its most obvious validation for this stand is the teaching that all young girls are the Virgin Mary's daughters, (Celeste Ashley, 2005).

The Jewish, Christian and Muslim faiths all attach considerable importance to premarital virginity, particularly that of women. Yet, the social valorization of virginity dates back to a much earlier time than the imposition of chastity upon unmarried women in Muslim communities. Neither the Koran nor Hadiths state that virginity is a precondition to marriage. Patriarchal societies aim to control the sexuality of women in order to regulate lines of descent and transfer. Islam has only translated a social into a religious norm. It is worth remembering that until the 1960s, moral and behavioral norms kept even European atheists from engaging in premarital sex. These constraints have been only gradually lifted in the last 50 years as a result of the liberalization of sexuality and the improved social status of women, (Jean-Jacques Amy, 2008).

The practice of virginity testing in Turkey has been in focus for long of advocacy on the part of women's human rights groups. In February 2002, Turkey issued a decree banning forced virginity testing following an announcement in July 2001 by the Turkish Health Minister that midwife and nursing students were required to be virgins, and that testing would be used to ensure compliance. Women in Turkish prisons are often subjected to compulsory, involuntary virginity testing immediately upon being incarcerated, and again prior to release, under the guise that virginity testing protects female prisoners. Virginity testing in South Africa claim that the practice is an effective method of preventing the spread of HIV and other sexually transmitted diseases as well as teenage pregnancies, (Kathambi Kinoti,2008).

In order to research the specifics of the Kosovo society and concepts associated with virginity we have analyzed virginity tests that are done at the Institute of Forensic Medicine in Prishtina and in term to compare conceptual differences with a category that is considered the most progressive and with a different vision we have made a survey among students in one public University and two private University College.

Virginity testing in Kosovo until the year 2002 was done by the order of the Court, prosecutor, police or social worker while after that this kind of testing is prohibited by law. However, being under strong pressure from interested parties in aim to avoid the problems that arise if such a test is done in private clinics in Kosovo, University Clinical Center established a professional committee composed by two gynecologists and one expert from forensic medicine which tests virginity on request by the interested parties. So, this is completely voluntary testing and mainly serves to resolve the problems between the partners, families involved or for confirmation of the state of hymen.

Anette Wickström from *Linköping University, in* Journal of the Royal Anthropological Institute, in 2010, presented virginity testing as the local people in Nkolokotho see it, as an urgent and vital necessity. In the face of a life-threatening epidemic, they are organizing something that is both a kind of local public health initiative and a collective ritual. If we are to analyze why people find it appropriate to act in this particular way, we need to understand the specific meanings of sexuality, integrity, and personhood found in the local community. However, people in Nkolokotho do not see virginity testing as a solution to the AIDS epidemic. In June 2005, the South African Parliament banned virginity testing for girls under the age of 16 (Children's Act 2005). Two months later, the newspapers reported that nearly 20,000 young women had visited the Zulu King's palace in Nongoma for the reed dance, to be tested and celebrate virginity for three days.

The period 2001-2010 was analyzed and it was found that during this time there were 544 virginity tests made. These tests are subjected to different categories of women, different ages, different reasons and with different social backgrounds.

Age of those who are subject of the test is different beginning from children, in three cases which have come at the insistence of the family with the aim of confirming the state of the hymen for reasons that are not described in the report. The predominant participant age was 25-35 years, age which relates to engagements and marriages between couples. Childhood and adolescence age appears very low, we have only 17 cases in age from 15-19 years and this information indicates that testing is not routine but women did it before or immediately after the beginning of sexual life.

The largest number of women who have sought to make the test belong to the category of "bachelor" neither married nor betrothed. This in our opinion best explained the reason why they are subject to this test. Half of the women in this category have made the test with their insistence and with the purpose of obtaining 'confirmation' that they are virgins. This phenomenon has its explanation in the fact that a significant number of women entering in relationship or even betrothed with Kosovo men's living in different western countries and virginity is a prerequisite required by men. Given that they don't know each other earlier by any means and they want their future partner to be a virgin, virginity test is key to create a safe relationship between them.

Another interesting finding is that all cases that are sent for testing by the prosecutor belong to this category of women that probably has to do with claims that were made for male partners of women who claimed to have been used only for sex and then they escaped. A part of the women form this category did the test after they declared the rape in prosecutor's office. A certain number of women has done the test in own will after a night spent with a male or after an unplanned sex being uncertain whether she is still a virgin or not. Married women take second place to the number of those who undergo testing and mainly after suspicion from their partner on the first night or first week of marriage.

Unfortunately in Kosovo there are still several locations in remote rural parts where the family insists to see the couple's blood stained bed sheet after the first night of marriage. There are times when they doubt that the female partner isn't a virgin and the divorce comes as a result of pressure from their family without sending a female for testing. In those cases, women go for testing in own will and receive confirmation of virginity which could help them to solve problems between them or their families. The same situation is with women's betrothed. There are cases after the start of a relationship when a doubt about virginity arises and the partner is one who insists that the test should be done before marriage because in this stage is much more easier to get a divorce if the woman isn't a virgin.

However, the decision of whether or not virginity is important depends essentially on personal choices. After all, a woman must be free to choose, without fear or coercion, what she can or cannot do to her own body.

Antony Kaminju wrote in BBC, 2007 *the article: South Africa's virginity testing*. He described how the girls feel after virginity test: "At 31 I'm very proud to be a virgin, and when I attend the test regularly it gives me self-esteem as a woman," said the nurse who works in the coastal city of Durban. Makhosaza June had been sending her 24-year-old daughter for virginity tests every month. "I have seen the effect on my daughter since she started attending the tests," she says. "She now has self-respect and she is the one who wants to attend those tests, I don't force her".

Knowing the difference between urban and rural area in their concepts dealing with the importance of female virginity we have analyzed the origin of women who underwent the test and their partners with particular emphasis to those who insist that by test can confirm that their partner is virgin or not. The difference between rural women and urban backgrounds has high significance. This significance is greater in the case of male partners who send their partners in testing. This difference is even greater when comparing the testing reasons in rural and urban area. The number of those who doubt on the partner's virginity is much higher in rural than urban area.

Suspicion expressed by partner is the main reason why women go for virginity testing. However, based in our study this is unreasonable because only 17% of the cases resulted in old broken hymen, 40% have been fresh broken, and 43% had intact hymen. Intact hymen phenomenon in this case can be explained with improper preparation of men for the first night of marriage and sex, elastic hymen or anteportas ejaculation which consequently results in the suspicion that their partner was not a virgin. This phenomena could be related to the old fashion view that if there "is no blood, there will be no marriage". Hard work needs to be done in this direction in terms of proper sexual education in the media, schools and community.

This phenomenon is quite disturbing because it causes unnecessary trauma in just married women or those who will soon enter into marriage.

For centuries, physicians have been called upon to determine whether or not a female is a 'virgin'. Yet, for practitioners without experience in the domain of pediatric and adolescent gynecology, it may be extremely difficult to differentiate between a healed, partial hymeneal tear and a naturally occurring superficial notch. In that age group, the hymen, being elastic, is not necessarily torn during coitus and even much less so on the occasion of sexual activities of a different type. Studies that specifically address how often the hymen tears following the first consensual penovaginal penetration are lacking. Among the complainants of sexual assault aged 14–19 years who stated that they were 'virgins' before the assault, only 19% had fresh hymeneal tears. Among 66 female complainants aged 15–64 years who denied coital experience prior to an alleged assault, only 9% had hymeneal tears. In some women without coital experience, the hymen is sufficiently distensible to allow a finger to be inserted into its opening, without rupturing,(Jean-Jacques,Amy,2008).

Abdul Kargbo, in 2008 wrote: "A court in Lille, France, annulled the marriage of a young engineer and a 20-year-old nursing student. The grounds for this annulment were not infidelity, violence, or even the ever-vague "irreconcilable differences." Rather, the marriage was dissolved because on the couple's wedding night in 2006, the groom had been unable to present a bloody sheet to the wedding guests who were partying downstairs. The groom apparently troubled by his inability to produce a bloody sheet—proof of his bride's virginity—went to court the next day and demanded an annulment. For her part, the new bride confessed to having sex before the wedding—presumably with someone other than her future husband".

The frequency of sexual relations between partners before virginity testing is analyzed in order to study a phenomenon in our society. We have to deal with the fact that most men do not have a clear vision about phenomenon of elastic hymen or anteportas ejaculation without possibility of penetration and hymen tear. In a lot of cases the partners claim to have had more than one sexual intercourse and the test result showed that the hymen is intact. In general, the most common outcome testing was intact hymen, 52.2% of all cases.

The study found evidence that the occupation of women who underwent the test belongs to the category of the unemployed and students. More than half of these women have proven to have intact hymen, the category of unemployed resulted to have more cases of fresh broken hymen when compared with those with old broken hymen while students had more cases with the old broken hymen. This is explained by the fact that unemployed women looking to find partners and entry into marriage are ready to do the test, receive confirmation and be ready to prove their virginity.

Considering the features of Kosovo society and the concept about virginity and the complicity associated with this issue, we prepared a self-administered questionnaire with specific questions dealing with attitudes of young people around this topic. This questionnaire, which was completely anonymous and confidential, was distributed among the students of the Public University in Kosovo and in a private University College.

The total number of respondents was approximately the same as the number of those who underwent virginity testing, 530 students in total. Gender representation was balanced, male 55.8% and 43.8% females. Their average age ranged 18-25 years, and their origin of residence was almost half and half, rural and urban

The first question which dealt with whether virginity is taboo topic, students answered with the significant difference that virginity is a taboo in Kosovo. There was no difference between sexes or student residence. This issue in our opinion is very worrying, especially having in mind that they should be the leaders of change and bring new concepts to this society which lives in conditions far above liberal. However, here again comes in place the major role of culture, tradition and religion in society. We think that their response has reflected the overall level of society and its concept about virginity and that this is not directly their opinion on this issue.

In 1918, continuing on from Totem and taboo and with the idea of finishing the series *Contributions to the psychology of love*, Freud wrote a short paper entitled *The taboo of virginity*. It is one of his works which is seldom commented upon; in any case, it is referred to far less often than the other two papers in the series. It would hardly be an exaggeration to say that it is a text which contemporary psychoanalysts have practically allowed to disappear into oblivion.

Giulia Sissa has shown, with plenty of evidence, that the Greeks, the Hippocratic physicians, the Romans and the early Church Fathers did not know of the existence of the hymen, in spite of their considerable knowledge of anatomy. Much later, physicians, freed of the ascendancy of theology, would re-establish this truth forgotten during the centuries of theocracy.

Elizabeth Day wrote in The Observer, 2008, that virginity is last taboo.

Advantage of being a virgin in Kosovo was confirmed in this study because regardless of gender, the majority of respondents claim that there is an advantage being virgin, with allusion that for a virgin girl it will be much easier to establish a relationship which will be crowned with marriage. One of our questions was if the virginity is a prerequisite for marriage and here we get an absolute answer yes to both sexes. These two answers show best the relationship between what is promoted as gender equality in society and factual position among the population. Although premarital sex life is pretty liberal in recent years in Kosovo, these statements indicate that young people deeply in their minds would rather marry a virgin.

The Shanghai Academy of Social Sciences surveyed 500 single men and women between 20 and 30 years old living in 25 neighborhoods. Researchers conducted the survey by sending out questionnaires and holding group discussions with students, blue- and white-collar workers and the unemployed. Nearly 41 percent of those surveyed were under the age of 22 and respondents were an almost equal mix of men and women. Nearly 60 percent said that virginity is one of the requirements for their ideal spouse - with both men and women saying they want to marry a virgin. Only 16.5 percent said they don't care about their partner's virginity.

When talking about virginity in Kosovo it means you are talking on female virginity. This was confirmed in this research because both genders overwhelmingly stated that female virginity isn't of the same importance as male virginity. The fact that nobody in the family or in society does not care if a man has had sexual affair before marriage does not apply to women, which if they lose virginity before marriage will face many problems, often being forced to undergo virginity testing and divorce which could have unforeseen consequences for the rest of her life. A divorced girl that was not a virgin on the first night of marriage, especially in rural areas and in patriarchal family has not a chance to marry a bachelor once more and her position in the family and society becomes more severe.

TalkAfrique, posted an article: Would you rather marry a virgin? In African perspective it was expected that a maiden must go into marriage as a virgin. If on the first night, her husband found her not to be so, the family suffered instant condemnation. But civilization has substantially changed the way people perceive virginity. At one time, it was even thought to be 'bush' if a girl dared reveal to her peers that she was still a virgin. Some girls even competed to be the first to lose their virginity to a boyfriend. Once again, attitudes are changing, and it is becoming fashionable to be a virgin. This new development is driven more by the Pentecostal revival spreading through the world. Virginity, at least among Pentecostal Christians and fundamentalist Muslims, is being appreciated again.

These findings presented above in the following question explain much better further conceptual difference between the sexes and inside society. On the question of whether you are virgin, 56% of respondents of both sexes answered no. The response among genders reveals that the number of virgin females is significantly greater, 61%, compared with men who are only 18%. Kosovo women's inferior position in this regard is confirmed in another question: would you marry a non virgin partner? Women overwhelmingly don't refuse to marry a non-virgin male and only 1/3 of men surveyed stated that they agree to marry a non-virgin female. It is interesting that among the students were not found significant differences between those who come from rural and urban areas.

The virginity rates among students at Wellesley College according to the student's major shows that: 0% of students with 'studio arts' major are virgins and Virginity rates for Spanish major (43%) is much lower than virginity rates for English and French majors (50%).

On Oldest and Largest Newspaper MIT's, sex survey we have found those data: 42 percent of students consider themselves virgins: 37 percent of men and 48 percent of women. The numbers are predictably higher for freshman class, which is 64 percent virgins: 60 percent of men and 69 percent of women.

Journal of Health Economics , 2008 published a paper by Sabia JJ: *The effect of adolescent virginity status on psychological well-being, using* data from the National Longitudinal Study of Adolescent Health to examine whether virginity status affects self-esteem and depression. For males, fixed effects and instrumental variables estimates provide little evidence that sex is causally related to psychological well-being. In contrast, estimates indicate that sexually active female adolescents are at increased risk of exhibiting the symptoms of depression relative to their counterparts who are not sexually active.

Mark Schuster et al. in their study: The Sexual Practices of Adolescent Virgins, published on American Journal of Public Health, took a survey of sexual risk of students in 9th through 12th grades in a socioeconomically diverse Los Angeles County school district in April 1992. They found out that 47% of the students were virgins. Virginity was more prevalent among those whose parents had higher education levels and who had higher educational expectations themselves.

Male respondents were asked directly about the virginity test because we were curios to get their opinion on this very sensitive issue. Although in preliminary questions had significant differences in between YES and NO response, giving absolute priority to being a virgin and virginity as a prerequisite for marriage, here a larger number responded that they would not seek to send their partners on virginity testing if they suspect that their partner is not virgin. Perhaps the fact that they have a greater sexual experience before marriage or their academic level did not leave them to freely express their opinion and result is such it is.

Maybe even most of them at the time of the survey are in a serious relationship with the partner they love and didn't think that something like this can happen is another reason that will actually be good to be true. When asked if the virginity test shows that the partner is not a virgin will result in divorce, we got equal claims received between those who say YES and those who will NOT divorce even if the test shows that the partner is not virgin. This answer, and this approach of young people gives hope in a near future with a little more work, education and openness to the world to make difference in the importance of female virginity and the need for virginity tests.

An opinion poll conducted by Information International for the American University of Beirut Medical Center, 2003, explored university students' perceptions on those issues and some of results are: More than half of the men polled in the survey said they would marry a non-virgin, with a breakdown by religion showing that 72.4% of Christian men had no problem with such an arrangement, compared with 45.8% of Muslim men. Out of those who would not agree to marry a non-virgin, the main reason cited was a lack of trust (75%), followed by religious considerations (62.5%), fear of STDs (54.7%), fear of family embarrassment (49.2%) and fear of social embarrassment (45.3%). In addition, 88.3% of males polled had heard of the procedure of hymeneal restoration, but only 25.7% of them approved of it. This is in comparison with 82% of women who were familiar with the procedure, out of which only 19.1% approved.

At the end of the survey, students were asked what they thought about hymen repair phenomenon that is widespread in recent times especially among women living in conservative society and which must necessarily be the virgin at the wedding night. In total the absolute answer was that hymenoplasty is not right action with the small difference from 5% between the sexes in favor of women's who prefer repair the hymen before marriage. This response is explained by the fact that still are some people who think that only hymen determines a female virginity and they are able to make such a action if necessary to obtain a marriage and a family in the future.

On the end it's important to put some phrase's circulated around about virginity: there is no way a virgin can be infected with STI's; a virgin can't have AIDS or HIV infection, which is transmitted by sexual interactions; there is no way a virgin can become pregnant; there is a lot of true love in virgin marriages; a woman who marries as a virgin rarely sees, or complains of problems as often as the non-virgin; it is difficult to find a virgin who has a problem getting married and usually at very early age which biology teaches is the optimal time for conception and establishing long and lasting relationship; virgins tend to be better prepared for marriage than non-virgins because of excitement; the non-virgins are worried about the future and have to make conscious effort to let their marriage work if they wish so; there is lot of fun and excitement for the virgin couple on wedding night; most men tend to respect virgins throughout their marriage vows.

It is a phenomenon that has exploded recently in Albania. It's about the operation which restores virginity. According to some statistics, which was published in "Osservatorio Balcani of Caucaso" paper, every day three Albanian girls undergo surgery to restore virginity.

These girls are from 18 to 30 years. They decide to present themselves as virgins to the man, with whom they would marry, throwing behind their past sexual relationships. They undergo this operation in secret.

For 20 minutes, females become virgin again. According to the report, the cost of such operation in public clinics is 200 Euros, while private ones are expensive. Director of maternity "Koco Gliozheni", Rubena Moisiu says that it is a complex phenomenon that plagues not only the girls who come from rural areas. Most of the operations, she says, are carried outin Tirana.

The reason of such operations, gynecologists and sociologists say, is the emigration of men abroad. They often come to find women to marry in their country. Virginity is a synonym of trust in the female partner and a good omen for the relationship

VII. CONCLUSIONS

- Virginity is still taboo in Kosovo,

- In Kosovo society there is still great controversy about virginity,

- Virginity testing is performed due to partners doubt, family insistence or with her own will, with women residing in rural areas being more representative in those cases,

- The main reason for virginity testing is partner doubt

- In more than half of cases, the test result has shown that the hymen is still intact and only a quarter of the cases have resulted with the old broken hymen,

- Female virginity is not the of the same importance as the male, being a virgin female is a priority and a prerequisite for marriage,

- Women would agree to marry a non- virgin partner and only 1/3 of the men declared that they would marry a non- virgin female,

- Half of men surveyed would not seek virginity test to determine whether their partner is virgin or not,

- Repairing the hymen is not preferred by young people in Kosovo,

- There is a need for a proper sexual and social education in order to reduce the need for virginity testing as a mean to prove female virginity which will be determining factor for the fate of many women in Kosovo society,

- There are weak signs that young people in Kosovo are starting to change the opinion about virginity.

VIII.REFERENCES

1. Abdul Kargbo: *No Blood-No Marriage or, Some Gentlemen Prefer Virgins,* T'Ings 'N Times, 2008

2. Anette Wickström: *Virginity testing as a local public health initiative: a 'preventive ritual' more than a 'diagnostic measure',* Journal of the Royal Anthropological Institute, 2010, 16: 532–550

3. Anke Bernau: *Virgins – a cultural history,* Granta Books, London, 2007

4. Annie Leah Sommers& Michael A. Sommers: *Virginity, Everything you need to know about,* The Rosen Publishing Group INC. New York, 2000

5. Anne Cloudsley: *Women of Omdurman, Life, Love and he Cult of Virginity,* St. Martin's Press Inc. 1984

6. Antony Kaminju: *South Africa's virginity testing,* BBC News, 2007

7. Alex Comfort, *The Yoy of Sex,* Pocket; 30 Anv edition , 2003

8. Bersamin MM, Fisher DA, Walker S, Hill DL, Grube JW: *Defining virginity and abstinence: adolescents' interpretations of sexual behaviors,* Adolesc Health. 2007 Aug;41(2):182-8

9. Carla Stephens: *A passion for Purity, Protecting God's Precious Gift of Virginity,* Harrison House, Oklahoma, 2003

10. Celeste Ashley: *How Different Cultures Handle Losing Their Virginity,* Isnare articles, 2005

11. Cubitt, C: *Virginity and Misogyny in Tenth- and Eleventh-Century England.* Gender & History, (2000), 12: 1–32

12. Cuong Manh La: *How virginity enhances masculinity: an exploratory study in Hanoi, Vietnam,* San Francisco State University, 2005

13. Dragoljub Zlatković:*Utvrđivanje nevinosti neveste u svadbenom ritual staroplaninskih sela,* Muzej Ponišavlja Pirot,30(2005) 3p.141-146

14. Elizabeth Landau: *What is virginity worth today?, CNN, 2009*

15. Hannah Bruckner, Peter Bearman: *After the promise: The STD consequences of adolescent virginity pledges,* Journal of Adolescent Health, Volume 36, Issue 4, P.271-278, April 2005

16. Higgins JA, Trussell J, Moore NB, Davidson JK: *Virginity lost, satisfaction gained? Physiological and psychological sexual satisfaction at heterosexual debut,* J Sex Res. 2010 Jul;47(4):384

17. Jean-Jacques Amy; *Certificates of virginity and reconstruction of the hymen,* The European Journal of Contraception and Reproductive Health Care June 2008;13(2):111–113

18. Joanne Stroud and Gail Thomas: *Images of the Untouched,* Dallas Spring Publications Inc. 1972

19. Judith A. Reisman& Edward W. Eichel: *Kinsey Sex and Fraud,* Lochinvar-Huntington House Publication, 1990

20. Katha Pollit: *Virginity or Death,* A Random House Trade Paperback Original, p224-226, USA, 2006

21. Kathambi Kinoti: *Virginity Testing and the War Against AIDS,* AWID - Association for Women's Rights in Development, 2008

22. Laura M. Carpenter: *Virginity Lost, An Intimate portrait of First Sexual Experiences*, New York University Press, 2005

23. Leonhard M. Weber: *On Marriage, Sex and Virginity*, Palm Publishers Montreal, 1966

24. Mary F. Foskett: *A Virgin Conceived*, Indian University Press, USA,2002

25. Martino SC, Elliott MN, Collins RL, Kanouse DE, Berry SH: *Virginity pledges among the willing: delays in first intercourse and consistency of condom use*, Adolescent Health. 2008 Oct;43(4):341-8

26. Melina M. Bersamin, Samantha Walker, Elizabeth D. Waiters, Deborah A. Fisher, and Joel W. Grube: *Promising to wait: virginity pledges and adolescent sexual behavior,* Journal of Adolescent Health 36 (2005) 428–436

27. Melina M. Bersamin, Deborah A. Fisher, Samantha Walker, Douglas L. Hill, and Joel W. Grube: *Defining virginity and abstinence: Adolescents' interpretations of sexual behaviors,* J Adolesc Health. 2007 August; 41(2): 182–188.

28. Mitike Molla, Yemane Berhane, Bernt Lindtjørn: *Traditional values of virginity and sexual behavior in rural Ethiopian youth: results from a cross-sectional study, BMC Public Health* 2008, 8:9

29. Ottokar Nemecek: *Virginity –Prenuptial rites and rituals*, The Citadel Press New York, 1962

30. Ramesh Adhikari and Jyotsna Tamang: *Premarital Sexual Behavior among male college students of Kathmandu, Nepal, BMC Public Health* 2009, 9:241

31. Raniero Cantalamessa: OFM Cap, *Virginity – A positive approach to celibacy for the Sake of the Kingdom of Heaven*, Alba House, New York, 1995

32. Robin Hanson: *Value of Virginity*, Overcoming Bias, 2007

33. Rosenbaum JE: *Patient teenagers? A comparison of the sexual behavior of virginity pledges and matched non-pledges,* Pediatrics. 2009 Jan;123(1):e110-20

34. Sabia JJ, Rees DI: *The effect of adolescent virginity status on psychological well-being,* J Health Econ. 2008 Sep;27(5):1368-81

35. Saint Augustine: *Marriage and Virginity*, New City Press, 1999

36. Sallie Foley, Sally A. Kope and Denis P. Sugrue: *Sex Matters for Woman*, The Guilford Press, New York, London, 2002

37. Serena Robar: *Giving up the V*, Simon Pulse, New York London Toronto Sydney, p3-10, 2009

38. Sithembile Promise Mhlongo: *Reasons for undergoing virginity testing: A study of young people in rural KwaZulu-Natal, South Africa*, University of KwaZulu-Natal, Durban, South Africa, 2009.

39. Skandrani S, Baubet T, Taïeb O, Rezzoug D, Moro MR: *The rule of virginity among young women of Maghrebine origin in France*, Transcult Psychiatry. 2010 Apr;47(2):301-13

40. T. G. Ramatsekisa: *The ban on virginity testing* ,Journal of US-China Public Administration, USA, Feb. 2010, Volume 7, No.2 (Serial No.52)

41. Vincent L; *Virginity testing in South Africa: re-traditioning the postcolony,* Cult Health Sex. 2006 Jan-Feb;8(1):17-30

42. Wickström, A. *Virginity testing as a local public health initiative: a 'preventive ritual' more than a 'diagnostic measure'.* Journal of the Royal Anthropological Institute, (2010), 16: 532–550

43. Women for Women's Human Rights/Kadinin Insan Halklari Projesi; *Turkey: Virginity examinations, 2001.*

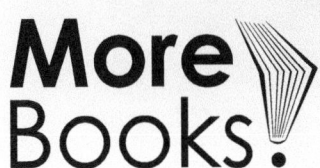
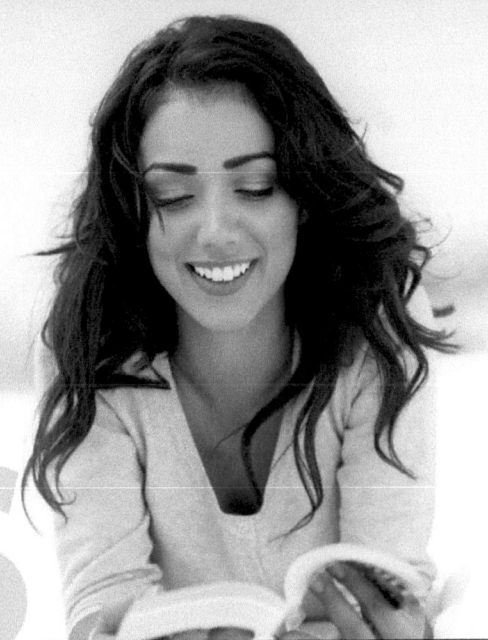

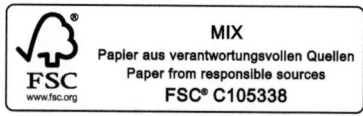
Printed by Books on Demand GmbH, Norderstedt / Germany